Dealing with ADHD:
Causes and Remedies

David Rex Orgen

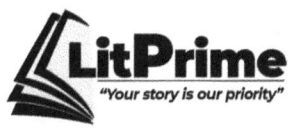

LitPrime
"Your story is our priority"

LitPrime Solutions
21250 Hawthorne Blvd
Suite 500, Torrance, CA 90503
www.litprime.com
Phone: 1-800-981-9893

Published by LitPrime Solutions: 04/24/2024

ISBN: 979-8-88703-356-3(sc)
ISBN: 979-8-88703-357-0(hc)
ISBN: 979-8-88703-358-7(e)

Library of Congress Control Number: 2024906549

Any people depicted in stock imagery provided by iStock are models, and such images are being used for illustrative purposes only.

Certain stock imagery © iStock.

Because of the dynamic nature of the Internet, any web addresses or links contained in this book may have changed since publication and may no longer be valid. The views expressed in this work are solely those of the author and do not necessarily reflect the views of the publisher, and the publisher hereby disclaims any responsibility for them.

Dedication

I dedicate this book to my amazing parents, especially my dad, who did not live to see me publish this book nor read it.

This book is also dedicated to all the incredible individuals living with disabilities, because all human beings are created equal.

TABLE OF CONTENTS

Acknowledgement

I would like to extend my heartfelt thanks and deepest gratitude to the numerous healthcare practitioners, county boards, and the entire community of persons with disabilities whom I've had the privilege to serve and listen to their incredible stories over the years.

I am profoundly grateful to everyone who has supported and cheered me on throughout my career.

Special acknowledgment goes to Rev. Richard Dunbar, a Retired Minister of the Capitol Area South District of the West Ohio Conference, who has been my mentor in the ministry. I am also indebted to Mrs. Jean Akyere Addison, MBA, Program Director of Mathlot Treatment Centre in Sacramento, California, for meticulously reading through the script, offering invaluable suggestions, and providing thoughtful insights.

Mrs. Sweetness Emma Danso, Founder of Oyemam Foundation and Advocate for Lupus awareness in Africa, deserves heartfelt appreciation for her review, valuable contributions, and inspiration which led me to write these books.

Pastor Bernard Adu-Danso of UMS, your contributions to this book are immensely appreciated.

To my family, especially my dear wife Sarah, your unwavering support and love mean the world to me. A special shout out to my children, David Sam, Daniel Albert, and Deborah Grace, who have consistently cheered me on.

INTRODUCTION

ADHD is not the "insignificant" disorder some imagine it to be. The direct "cost of illness" associated with ADHD across all ages in the US is estimated to be over $74 billion (using conservative incidence rates estimates). In 2013, a study found that the total spending on ADHD cases ranged from $143 billion to $266 billion a year, and the direct annual costs for treatment were estimated to be $1,574 per person, plus $2,278 a year for family members when indirect costs like productivity losses were taken into account

Although ADHD does not have a cure, it can be successfully managed with therapy to bring out the best in individuals. There are many successful individuals who have attained great heights of success in business, arts, sports and other endeavours regardless of their ADHD diagnoses.

This book seeks to show you what ADHD is all about and

how to live a well-fulfilled life not only for the ADHD diagnosed person but also for the parent, guardian, or supporting family member.

CHAPTER

1

What is ADHD?

Attention-Deficit/Hyperactivity Disorder (ADHD) is a brain disorder marked by an ongoing pattern of inattention and/or hyperactivity-impulsivity that interferes with functioning or development.[2] Nearly every mainstream medical, psychological, and educational organisation in the United States long ago concluded that ADHD is a real, brain-based medical disorder.[1] It is a non-discriminatory disorder affecting people of every age, gender, IQ, religious, and socio-economic background.

Inattention

This means a person wanders off tasks, lacks persistence, has difficulty sustaining focused, and is disorganised; these problems are not due to defiance or lack of comprehension.

Hyperactivity

This means a person seems to move about constantly, even in situations in which it is not appropriate. When it is not appropriate, the person excessively fidgets, taps, or talks. In adults, it may be extreme restlessness or wearing others out with their activity.

Impulsivity

Where a person makes hasty actions that occur at the moment without first thinking about the actions and that may be potentially harmful; a desire for immediate rewards or an inability to delay gratification. An impulsive person may be socially intrusive and excessively interrupt others or make important decisions without considering the long-term consequences.

ADHD is not benign. [1] However, when the ADHD is undiagnosed and untreated, ADHD contributes to:

- Problems succeeding in school and successfully graduating.

- Problems at work, lost productivity, and reduced earning power.

- Problems with relationships.

- More driving citations and accidents.

- Problems with overeating and obesity.

- Problems with the law.

ADHD is NOT caused by moral failure, poor parenting, family problems, poor teachers or schools, too much TV, food allergies, or excess sugar. Instead, research shows that ADHD is both highly genetic, with the majority of ADHD cases having a genetic component, and a brain-based disorder, with the symptoms of ADHD linked to many specific brain areas. [1]

CHAPTER

2

Prevalence

ADHD is one of the most common neurodevelopment disorders of childhood. It is usually first diagnosed in childhood and often lasts into adulthood.

Although there is no global consensus on the prevalence of attention-deficit/hyperactivity disorder (ADHD) in children, adolescents, and adults, metaregression analyses have estimated the worldwide prevalence at between 5.29% and 7.1% in children and adolescents, and at 3.4% (range 1.2–7.3%) in adults. The prevalence of ADHD in very young children (aged <6 years) or later in adult life (aged >44 years) is less well-studied.[2]

Prevalence Factors

ADHD prevalence rates may vary depending on several factors:

Age – Whilst ADHD was once considered to be a childhood disease with a decline in symptoms during maturation into adulthood, it is now acknowledged to persist into adulthood in an estimated 50–66% of individuals.

Gender – A higher prevalence of ADHD is often reported in males.

Presentations of ADHD – The combined inattentive-hyperactive-impulsive presentation of ADHD is considered most prevalent in children, adolescents, and adults. [2]

ADHD is often present alongside comorbidities such as oppositional defiant disorder, conduct disorder, anxiety disorder, personality disorders and depression, which may further complicate understanding of true prevalence rates.

Children

According to new research, about 7% of children worldwide have ADHD. This estimate, which differs significantly from other appraisals, is based on data from 175 prior studies conducted over nearly four decades. [6]

This estimate comes in lower than the latest data from the U.S. Centers for Disease Control and Prevention, which reports that 11% of U.S. school-age children had been diagnosed with ADHD by 2011.

In a new study, published online in Pediatrics, the researchers combed through decades' worth of research on ADHD and identified 175 studies with 179 estimates of ADHD prevalence. When aggregated, the results contained data collected from over 1 million children over a 36-year period. These studies were conducted in North America and Europe.

According to the report, all that data added up to a worldwide ADHD estimate of 7.2%, with a range running from 6.7% to 7.8%. [6]

ADHD On The Rise

Cases and diagnoses of ADHD have been increasing dramatically in the past few years. While the American Psychiatric Association (APA) says that 5% of American children have ADHD, the Centers for Disease Control and Prevention (CDC) puts the number at more than double the APA's number. According to the CDC, 11% of American children, ages 4 to 17, have attention disorders. This reflects an increase of 42% in just eight years.[5]

Increase in Diagnoses:

- 2003: 7.8%

- 2007: 9.5%

- 2011: 11 %

As mentioned in the previous paragraph, the percentage of children estimated to have ADHD has changed over time. A historical view provides the necessary context to understand changes in what we know about ADHD. This includes estimates of the rates of ADHD across time, changes in diagnostic criteria, and the evolution of medication treatment.

Children

Recent surveys show that:

- Approximately 11% of children (6.4 million) aged 4-17 years were diagnosed with ADHD as of 2011. This means 11 out of every 100 children or not less than 1 out of 10 children, will receive a diagnosis of ADHD.[4]

- Rates of ADHD diagnosis increased by an average of approximately 5% per year from 2003 to 2011. Boys (13.2%) were more likely than girls (5.6%) to have ever been diagnosed with ADHD.[4]

- The average age of ADHD diagnosis was 7 years, but children reported by their parents to have had more severe ADHD were diagnosed earlier. [4]

Adults

Estimates from individual studies have indicated that the global prevalence of ADHD in adults ranges from 1.1% in Australia to 7.3% in France (see Figure 1).[2]

Prevalence of ADHD in adults by country

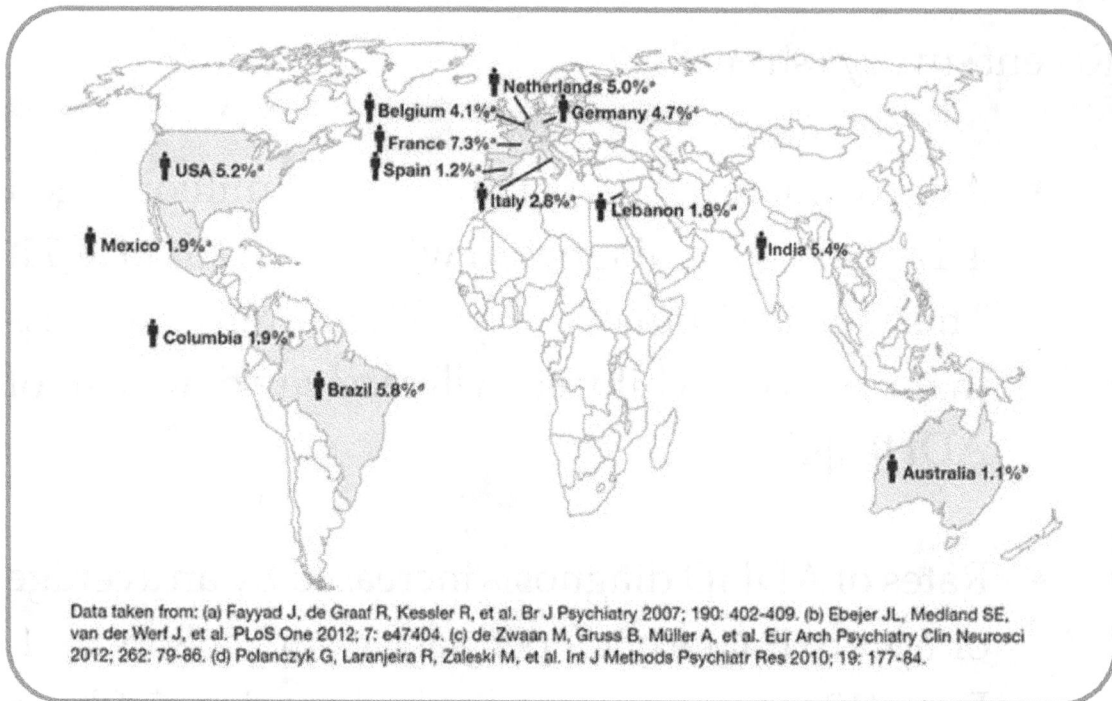

Data taken from: (a) Fayyad J, de Graaf R, Kessler R, et al. Br J Psychiatry 2007; 190: 402-409. (b) Ebejer JL, Medland SE, van der Werf J, et al. PLoS One 2012; 7: e47404. (c) de Zwaan M, Gruss B, Müller A, et al. Eur Arch Psychiatry Clin Neurosci 2012; 262: 79-86. (d) Polanczyk G, Laranjeira R, Zaleski M, et al. Int J Methods Psychiatr Res 2010; 19: 177-84.

Nevertheless, review papers have concluded that ADHD prevalence data may vary widely between studies due to various factors such as population characteristics; methodological differences, environmental and cultural variations, and variability in identification and diagnostic guideline tools employed in studies, rather than geographical location.

Medication Treatment

Research shows that, currently, 6.1% of all American children are being treated for ADHD with medication.

Some states have higher rates of treatment with medication than others. In spite of this, one in five American children who have been diagnosed with ADHD is not receiving medicine or mental health counselling for their disorder.

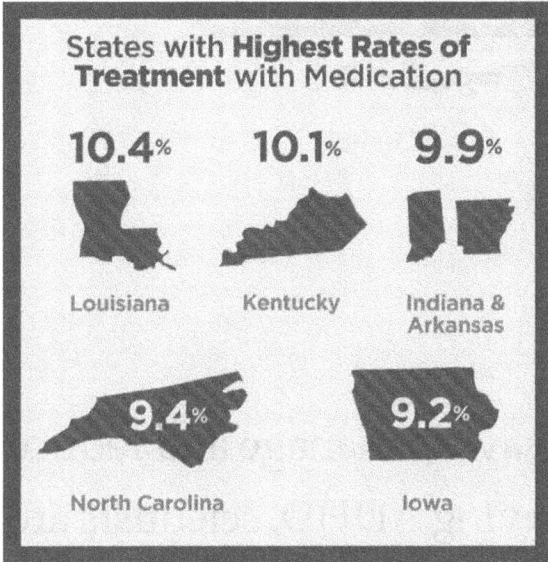

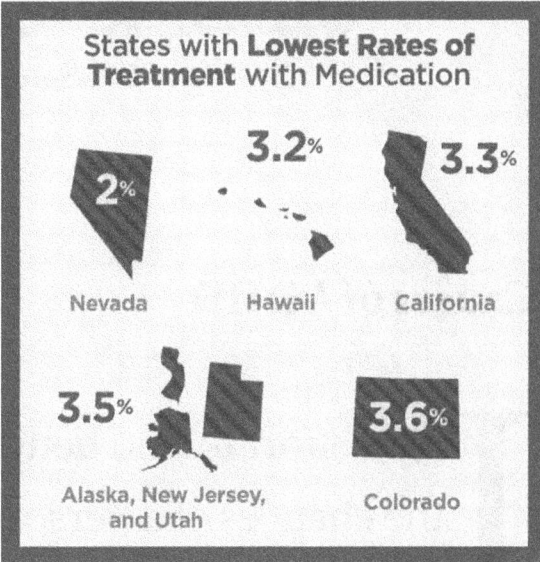

States with **Highest Rates of Treatment** with Medication

10.4% Louisiana

10.1% Kentucky

9.9% Indiana & Arkansas

9.4% North Carolina

9.2% Iowa

States with **Lowest Rates of Treatment** with Medication

2% Nevada

3.2% Hawaii

3.3% California

3.5% Alaska, New Jersey, and Utah

3.6% Colorado

CHAPTER

3

Causes and Risk Factors

Causes of ADHD

In an effort to find better ways to manage and reduce the chances of a person having ADHD, scientists are continuously studying the causes and risk factors. The cause(s) of ADHD are unknown, but current research shows that genetics plays an important role.

Research does not support the popularly held views that ADHD is caused by eating too much sugar, watching too much television, parenting, or social and environmental factors such as poverty or family chaos. While these factors may exacerbate symptoms, particularly in certain individuals, the evidence is not strong enough to conclude that they are the primary causes of ADHD

Risk Factors

Though it is not certain what causes ADHD, like many other illnesses, a number of factors can contribute to ADHD, such as:

- Genes
- Cigarette smoking, alcohol use, or drug use during pregnancy
- Exposure to environmental toxins during pregnancy
- Exposure to environmental toxins, such as high levels of lead, at a young age
- Low birth weight
- Brain injuries

ADHD is more common in males than females, and females with ADHD are more likely to have problems primarily with inattention. Additionally, other conditions, such as learning disabilities, anxiety disorder, conduct disorder, depression, and substance abuse, are common in people with ADHD.

Demographics

There are demographic factors that impact the risks of being diagnosed with ADHD.

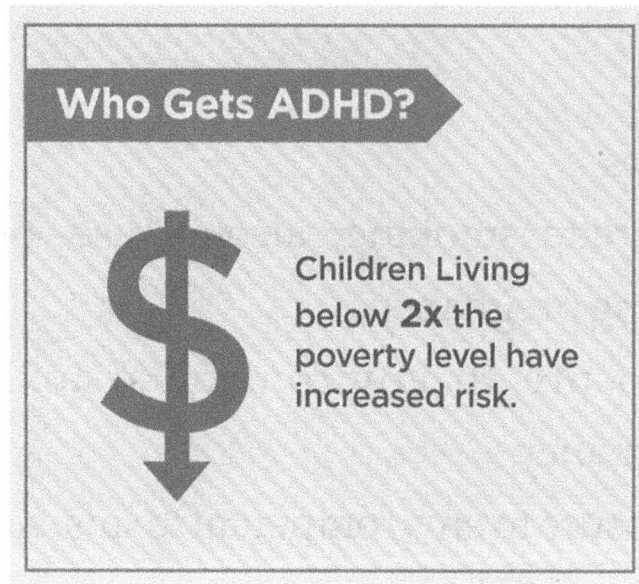

Who Gets ADHD?

$ Children Living below **2x** the poverty level have increased risk.

Children living in households that make less than twice the federal poverty level have a higher risk of being diagnosed with ADHD compared to children from higher-income households.

Race

Certain conditions might affect individuals of different

races in different ways, but ADHD impacts children of all races.

The prevalence of ADHD in children, broken down by race, is as follows:

- Whites: 9.8%
- Blacks: 9.5%
- Latinos: 5.5%

CHAPTER

4

Symptoms and Diagnosis

Symptoms

People with ADHD may have trouble paying attention, controlling impulsive behaviours (acting without considering the consequences), or be hyperctive. Although ADHD can't be cured, it can be successfully managed, and some symptoms may improve as the child ages.

Symptoms in Children

It is normal for children to have trouble focusing and behaving at one time or another. However, children with ADHD do not simply grow out of these behaviours. The symptoms continue and can lead to challenges at school, at home, or with friends.

A child with ADHD might:

- Daydream a lot
- Forget or lose things frequently
- Squirm or fidget
- Talk excessively
- Make careless mistakes or take unnecessary risks
- Have a hard time resisting temptation
- Struggle with taking turns
- Have difficulty getting along with others

In preschool children, the most common ADHD symptom is hyperactivity.

It is normal to have some inattention, unfocused motor activity, and impulsivity. For people with ADHD, these behaviours:

- Are more severe,
- Occur more often, and
- Interfere with or reduce the quality of how they function socially, at school, or in a job

Symptoms Varying with Sex

Boys and girls exhibit very different ADHD symptoms, with boys being more likely to be diagnosed with the attention disorder.

Why? The nature of ADHD symptoms in boys makes their condition more noticeable than in girls.

Boys tend to display externalised symptoms that most people think of when they think of ADHD behaviour, for example:

- Impulsivity or "acting out"
- Hyperactivity; such as running and hitting
- Lack of focus; including inattentiveness
- Physical aggression

Boys and girls display very different ADHD symptoms.

Boys' symptoms are obvious and "external":

$%#!

- Impulsivity or "acting out"
- Hyperactivity, such as running and hitting
- Lack of focus, including inattentiveness
- Physical aggression

Girls' symptoms are less obvious, and more "internal":

- Being withdrawn
- Low self-esteem and anxiety
- Intellectual impairment and difficulty with academic achievement
- Inattentiveness or a tendency to "daydream"
- Verbal aggression: teasing, taunting, or namecalling

ADHD in girls is often easy to overlook because it is not "typical" ADHD behaviour. The symptoms are not as obvious as they are in boys. They can include:

- Being withdrawn
- Low self-esteem and anxiety
- Intellectual impairment and difficulty with academic achievement
- Inattentiveness or a tendency to "daydream"
- Verbal aggression; teasing, taunting, or name-calling

Diagnosis

For a person to receive a diagnosis of ADHD, the symptoms of inattention and/or hyperactivity-impulsivity must be chronic or long-lasting, impair the person's functioning, and cause the person to fall behind normal development for his or her age. Thus, deciding if a child has ADHD is a several-step process that requires a comprehensive evaluation by a licensed clinician, such as a paediatrician, psychologist, or psychiatrist with expertise in ADHD.

There is no single test to diagnose ADHD, and many other problems, like anxiety, depression, and certain types of learning disabilities, can have similar symptoms. One step of the process involves having a medical exam, including hearing and vision tests, to rule out other problems with symptoms like ADHD. Another part of the process may include a checklist for rating ADHD symptoms and taking a history of the child from parents, teachers, and sometimes, the child.

The doctor will also ensure that any ADHD symptoms are not due to another medical or psychiatric condition. Most children with ADHD receive a diagnosis during their elementary school years. For an adolescent or adult to receive a diagnosis of ADHD, the symptoms need to have been present prior to age 12.

ADHD symptoms can appear as early as between the ages of 3 and 6 years and can continue through adolescence and adulthood.

> *Symptoms of ADHD can be mistaken for emotional or disciplinary problems or missed entirely in quiet, well-behaved children, leading to a delay in diagnosis.*

Adults with undiagnosed ADHD may have a history of poor academic performance, problems at work, or difficult and failed relationships.

ADHD symptoms can change over time as a person ages.

In young children with ADHD, hyperactivity-impulsivity is the most predominant symptom. As a child reaches elementary school, the symptoms of inattention may become more prominent and cause the child to struggle academically. In adolescence, hyperactivity seems to lessen and may manifest more often as feelings of restlessness or fidgeting, but inattention and impulsivity may remain. Many adolescents with ADHD also grapple with relationship challenges and antisocial behaviours. Inattention, restlessness, and impulsivity tend to persist into adulthood.

Time of Diagnoses

Children are diagnosed at different ages and detecting symptoms differs from case to case. Generally, the more severe the symptoms, the earlier the diagnosis tends to occur.

The following are examples of the average age of diagnosis for children with ADHD:

- 8 years old: average age of diagnosis for children with mild ADHD

- 7 years old: average age of diagnosis for children with moderate ADHD

- 5 years old: average age of diagnosis for children with severe ADHD

CHAPTER

5

Types & Therapy

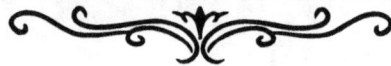

Types

There are three different types of ADHD, depending on which types of symptoms are strongest in the individual. They are Predominantly Inattentive Presentation, Predominantly Hyperactive-Impulsive Presentation, and Combined Presentation.

Predominantly Inattentive Presentation

People with symptoms of inattention may often:

- Overlook or miss details, make careless mistakes in schoolwork, at work, or during other activities

- Have problems sustaining attention in tasks or during play, including conversations, lectures, or lengthy reading

- Not seem to listen when spoken to directly;

- Not follow through on instructions and fail to finish schoolwork, chores, or duties in the workplace or start tasks but quickly lose focus and get easily sidetracked

- Have problems organising tasks and activities, such as what to do in sequence, keeping materials and belongings in order, having messy work and poor time management, and failing to meet deadlines

- Avoid or dislike tasks that require sustained mental effort, such as schoolwork or homework, or for teens and older adults, preparing reports, completing forms, or reviewing lengthy papers

- Lose things necessary for tasks or activities, such

as school supplies, pencils, books, tools, wallets, keys, paperwork, eyeglasses, and cell phones

- Be easily distracted by unrelated thoughts or stimuli

- Be forgetful in daily activities, such as chores, errands, returning calls, and keeping appointments

- It is hard for the individual, to pay attention to details

- The person is easily distracted or forgets details of daily routines

Predominantly Hyperactive-Impulsive Presentation

People with symptoms of hyperactivity-impulsivity may often:

- Fidget and squirm in their seats

- Leave their seats in situations when staying seated is expected, such as in the classroom or in the office

- Run or dash around or climb in situations where it is inappropriate or, in teens and adults, often feel restless

- Be unable to play or engage in hobbies quietly

- Be constantly in motion or "on the go," or act as if "driven by a motor"

- Talk nonstop

- Blurt out an answer before a question has been completed or finish other people's sentences

- Have trouble waiting their turn

- Interrupt or intrude on others, for example in conversations, games, or activities

- The individual feels restless and has trouble with impulsivity.

- Someone who is impulsive may interrupt others a lot, grab things from people, or speak at inappropriate times.

- It is hard for the person to wait their turn or listen to directions. A person with impulsivity may have more accidents and injuries than others.

Combined Presentation

- Symptoms of the two types above are present in the person. As symptoms can change over time, the presentation may change over time as well.

Therapy

ADHD & Other Conditions

ADHD doesn't increase a person's risk for other conditions or diseases. However, some people with ADHD — especially children — are more likely to experience a range of co-existing conditions. They can sometimes make social situations more difficult or school more challenging.

Some co-existing conditions include:

- Conduct disorders and difficulties, including anti-social behaviour, fighting, and oppositional defiant disorder
- Anxiety disorder
- Depression
- Bipolar disorder
- Tourette's syndrome
- Substance abuse
- Learning disabilities
- Bed-wetting problems
- Sleep disorders

Treatment and Therapies

In most cases, ADHD is best treated with a combination of behaviour therapy and medication. For preschool-aged children (4-5 years of age) with ADHD, behaviour therapy is recommended as the first line of treatment. No single treatment is the answer for every child and good treatment plans will include close monitoring, follow-ups, and any needed changes made along the way.

While there is no cure for ADHD, currently available treatments, which include medication, psychotherapy, education or training, or a combination of treatments, can help reduce symptoms and improve functioning.

Medication

For many people, ADHD medications reduce hyperactivity and impulsivity and improve their ability to focus, work, and learn. Medication may also improve physical coordination. Sometimes several different medications or dosages must be tried before finding the right one that works for a particular person. Anyone taking medications must be monitored closely and carefully by their prescribing doctor.

Stimulants

The most common type of medication used for treating ADHD is called a "stimulant." Although it may seem unusual to treat ADHD with a medication that is considered a stimulant, it works because it increases the brain chemicals dopamine and norepinephrine, which play essential roles in thinking and attention.

Under medical supervision, stimulant medications are considered safe. However, there are risks and side effects, especially when they are misused or taken in excess of the prescribed dose. For example, stimulants can raise blood pressure and heart rate and increase anxiety. Therefore, a person with other health problems, including high blood pressure, seizures, heart disease, glaucoma, liver or kidney disease, or an anxiety disorder should tell their doctor before taking a stimulant.

Talk with a doctor if you see any of these side effects while taking stimulants:

- Decreased appetite
- Sleep problems
- Tics (sudden, repetitive movements or sounds); personality changes
- Increased anxiety and irritability
- Stomachaches
- Headaches

Non-stimulants

A few other ADHD medications are non-stimulants. These medications take longer to start working than stimulants, but can also improve focus, attention, and impulsivity in a person with ADHD. Doctors may prescribe a non-stimulant: when a person has bothersome side effects from stimulants; when a stimulant was not effective; or in combination with a stimulant to increase effectiveness.

Although not approved by the U.S. Food and Drug Administration (FDA) specifically for the treatment of ADHD, some antidepressants are sometimes used alone or in combination with a stimulant to treat ADHD. Antidepressants may help with all of the symptoms of ADHD and can be prescribed if a patient has bothersome side effects from stimulants. Antidepressants can be helpful in combination with stimulants if a patient also has another condition, such as an anxiety disorder, depression, or another mood disorder.

In my experience as a non-clinical home healthcare provider, I have collaborated with my patients on numerous occasions to identify the most effective medication, dosage, or combination of medications.

Psychotherapy

Adding psychotherapy to ADHD treatment can help patients and their families to better cope with everyday problems.

Behavioural Therapy is a type of psychotherapy that aims to help a person change their behaviour. It might involve practical assistance, such as help with organising tasks or completing schoolwork, or working through emotionally difficult events.

Behavioural therapy also teaches a person how to:

- Monitor their own behaviour
- Give oneself praise or rewards for acting in a desired way, such as controlling anger or thinking

before acting.

Parents, teachers, and family members also can give positive or negative feedback for certain behaviours and help establish clear rules, chore lists, and other structured routines to help a person control their behaviour. Therapists may also teach children social skills, such as how to wait their turn, share toys, ask for help, or respond to teasing. Learning to read facial expressions and the tone of voice in others, and how to respond appropriately can also be part of social skills training.

Cognitive Behavioural Therapy

This involves teaching a person mindfulness techniques, or meditation. A person learns how to be aware and accepting of one's thoughts and feelings to improve focus and concentration. The therapist also encourages the person with ADHD to adjust to some life changes that come with treatment, such as thinking before acting or resisting the urge to take unnecessary risks.

Family and Marital Therapy

This can help family members and spouses find better ways to handle disruptive behaviours, encourage behaviour changes, and improve interactions with the patient.

Education and Training:

Children and adults with ADHD need guidance and understanding from their parents, families, and teachers to reach their full potential and to succeed. For school-age children, frustration, blame, and anger may have built up within a family before a child is diagnosed. Parents and children may need special help to overcome negative feelings. Mental health professionals can educate parents about ADHD and how it affects a family. They will also help the child and their parents develop new skills, attitudes, and ways of relating to each other.

Parenting Skills Training (Behavioural Parent Management Training)

This teaches parents the skills they need to encourage and reward positive behaviours in their children. It helps parents learn how to use a system of rewards and consequences to change a child's behaviour. Parents are taught to give immediate and positive feedback for behaviours they want to encourage and ignore or redirect behaviours that they want to discourage. They may also learn to structure situations in ways that support desired behaviour.

Stress Management Techniques

This can benefit parents of children with ADHD by increasing their ability to deal with frustration so that they can respond calmly to their child's behaviour.

Support Groups

This can help parents and families connect with others who have similar problems and concerns. Groups often meet regularly to share frustrations and successes, exchange information about recommended specialists and strategies, and talk with experts.

Tips to Help Children and Adults with ADHD Stay Organised

For Kids:

For Children, parents and teachers can help kids with ADHD stay organized and follow directions with tools such as:

Keeping a routine and a schedule

Maintain the same routine every day, from wake-up time to bedtime. Include dedicated times for homework, outdoor play, and indoor activities. Keep the schedule on the refrigerator or a bulletin board in the kitchen. Make sure to write changes on the schedule as far in advance as possible.

Organizing everyday items

Have a specific place for everything, and keep everything in its place. This includes clothing, backpacks, toys, etc.

Using homework and notebook organisers

Use organisers for school materials and supplies. Emphasize to your child the importance of writing down assignments and ensuring they bring home the necessary books.

Being clear and consistent

Children with ADHD need consistent rules they can understand and follow.

Giving praise or rewards when rules are followed

Children with ADHD often receive and expect criticism. Look for good behaviour, and praise it.

For Adults:

A professional counsellor or therapist can help an adult with ADHD learn how to organise their life with tools such as:

Keeping routines

Making lists for different tasks and activities Using a calendar for scheduling events

Using reminder notes

Assigning a special place for keys, bills, and paperwork Breaking down large tasks into more manageable, smaller steps so that completing each part of the task provides a sense of accomplishment.

CHAPTER

6

Social and Economic Impact

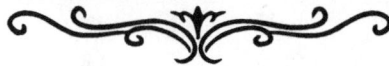

Attention-Deficit/Hyperactivity Disorder (ADHD) is associated with increased healthcare costs for people of all ages with the disorder. These costs may be attributed to medication expenses, loss of income from unemployment, increased incidence of accidents, and potential substance abuse issues.

Medical Costs

Cost is a major factor when it comes to how a condition affects someone. Treatment plans and medications can be expensive, and planning around payment can be stressful.

How Much Does It Cost?

$14,576 — Average cost of ADHD per person

Yearly cost to Americans — **$42.5 Billion**

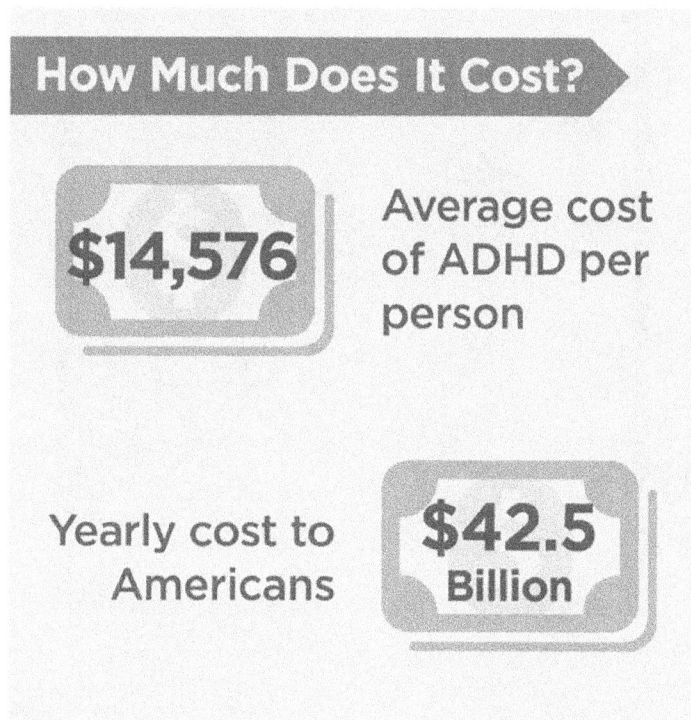

A study from 2007 claimed that the "cost of illness" for a person with ADHD is $14,576 each year. This implies that ADHD costs Americans $42.5 billion each year — and that's on the conservative side. [5]

Related Expenses

Medicines and treatments are not the only costs to consider when dealing with an ADHD diagnosis.

Other factors that can make a dent in your pocketbook include:

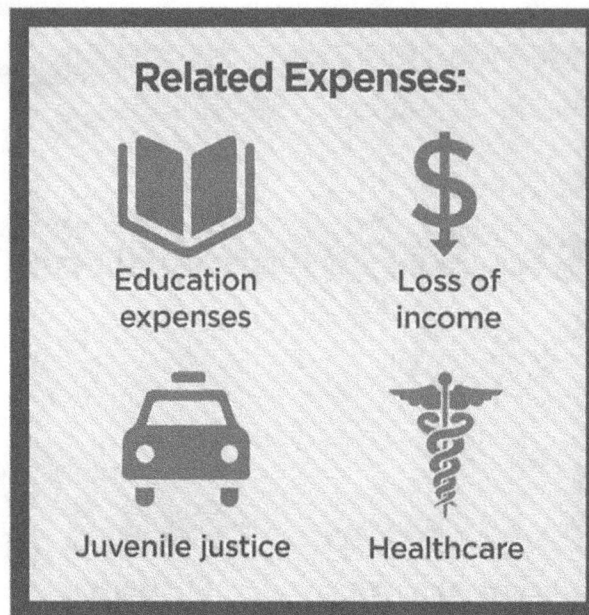

- Education expenses
- Loss of work
- Juvenile justice
- Healthcare costs

Healthcare Resource Use

A major contributory factor to the societal burden of ADHD is the increased healthcare resource use observed in patients with ADHD.

In a German study conducted in 2008, 30,264 patients were diagnosed with ADHD, with a mean total cost of €3,888 per patient in that year. This included incremental costs of €2,902 per patient in that year, which were mostly due to therapeutic devices and remedies like occupational therapy.

In the UK, estimated annual healthcare costs associated with the treatment of ADHD in adolescents have been reported as £670 million, with education and National Health Service (NHS) resources accounting for approximately 76% and 24% of spending, respectively. In 2010, this equated to a mean cost per adolescent for NHS, social care, and education resources of £5493. [5]

Canada loses an estimated $6 billion to $11 billion annually through loss of workplace productivity.

National ADHD-related costs (in millions) by cost categories in Europe using the Netherlands as a reference case. [2]

€161 M
(11 %)

€377 M
(25 %)

€84 M
(8 %)

€161 M
(15 %)

€339 M
(22 %)

€143 M
(14 %)

€4.3 M
(0.4 %)

€4.3 M
(0.3 %)

€648 M
(62 %)

€648 M
(42 %)

Healthcare (patient)

Education (patient)

Social services (patient)

Productivity losses (family member)

Healthcare (family member)

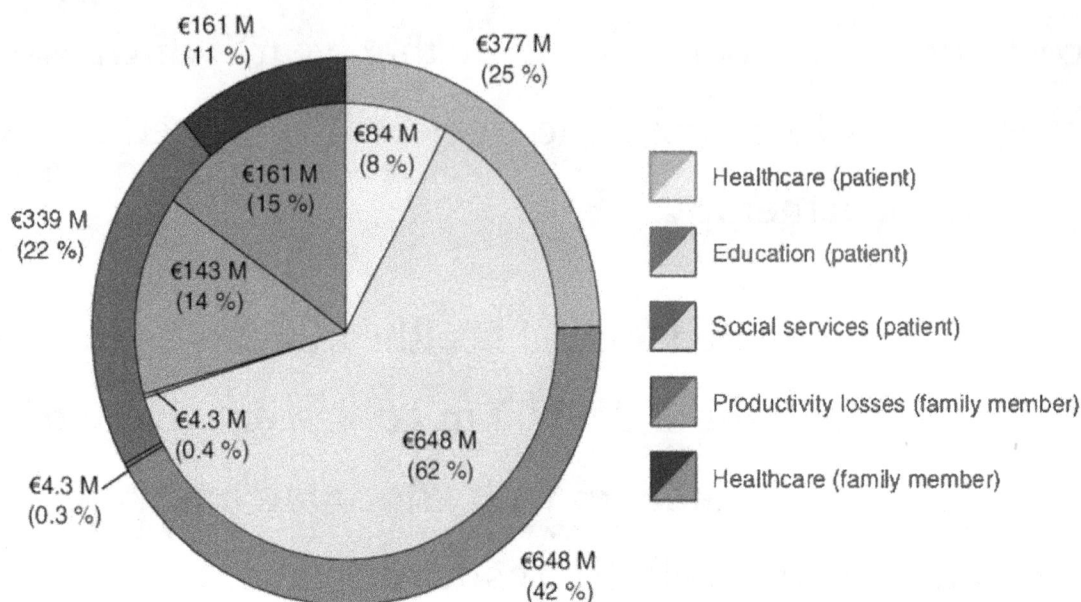

A retrospective analysis of healthcare claims in the US found that for over five years, there were 150,936 adults with at least one ADHD-related claim. Overall, adults with ADHD incurred a higher total healthcare expenditure compared with adults without ADHD.

Furthermore, a US study found that elevated healthcare resource use may reflect the increased rate of injuries observed in patients with ADHD. In a study of adults enrolled in an employer-sponsored health plan, injury claims were more common in individuals with ADHD than in non-ADHD controls (21.5% vs 15.7%).

Burden to Individuals and Employers

ADHD carries a burden in terms of absenteeism from the workplace. A study conducted by the World Health Organisation in 10 countries across Europe and the Americas reported that workers with ADHD had 22.1 more days of annual absenteeism compared with employees without the disorder. [2]

Financial difficulties may thus arise for adults with ADHD if they are unable to retain steady employment.

In a US study, adults with self-reported ADHD were less likely to be employed (either full-time or part-time), more likely to be looking for work, and reported changing jobs more frequently in the previous 10 years, compared with controls.

Employment status among US adults aged 18–64 years with self-reported ADHD. [2]

	ADHD	Non - ADHD
Employed	52%***	72%
Employed full-time	34%***	57%
Looking for work	14%***	5%
Mean number of jobs held over previous 10 years	5.4***	3.4

Furthermore, a series of European and North American focus groups found that 49% of adults with ADHD experienced problems with finances and spending.

Additionally, there is some evidence that parents or caregivers of children with ADHD may experience financial difficulties, thus impacting the entire family.

One study in the Netherlands found that the mean annual indirect cost due to absence from work and reduced efficiency at work was more than three-fold higher for mothers of children with ADHD (£2,243), compared with those who had children with or without other behavioural problems (£408 and £674, respectively). [2]

A study in the US found that adults with ADHD had significantly higher absence days (9 vs 7) and higher turnover (9% vs 5%) compared with adults without ADHD. Similar results were also found for caregivers of children with ADHD in comparison to caregivers of children without ADHD, with absence days at 8 vs 7; and turnover at 5% vs 4%, respectively. [2]

Health Care

- Immediate costs of increased general medical expenses, accidents, and emergency room visits.

- Long-term costs of higher rates of mental health illness, substance use and abuse including alcohol and cigarettes, increased driving accidents, earlier and riskier sexual activity, and increased medical costs to family members.

Education

- Students with ADHD are at a higher risk for lower academic achievement, grade retention, special education, disciplinary referrals, and dropping out of high school.

Justice and Correction

- Incidence rates of criminal activity are far greater for those with ADHD; offending begins earlier and there are higher rates of recidivism.

Social Services

- Those with ADHD have a greater period of unemployment and are more dependent on social welfare.

Peer Relationships

- Parents of children with a history of ADHD report almost 3 times as many peer problems as those without a history of ADHD (21.1% vs. 7.3%).

- Parents report that children with a history of ADHD are almost 10 times as likely to have difficulties that interfere with friendships (20.6% vs. 2.0%).

Injury

- A higher percentage of parents of children with attention-deficit/hyperactivity disorder reported non-fatal injuries (4.5% vs. 2.5% for healthy children).

- Children with ADHD, compared to children without ADHD, were more likely to have major injuries (59% vs. 49%), hospital inpatient admissions (26% vs. 18%), hospital outpatient admissions (41% vs. 33%), or emergency department admission (81% vs. 74%).

- Data from international samples suggest that young people with high levels of attentional difficulties are at greater risk of involvement in a motor vehicle crashes, drinking and driving, and traffic violations.

CHAPTER

7

Success Story

Narrated by a mother with ADD

After half a lifetime of struggling at home and work and dreading each new day, I feel as though a new me has been born with my adult ADD diagnosis.

I'm sitting in the tiny nurses' station, staring at neat piles of completed paperwork. It's only 1:30 a.m. and I'm done already. Work that used to have me scrambling to finish before the day-shift nurse came in at 7 a.m. was completed. Not just completed, done right, with a clear focus.

I smile, leaning back in my chair. So this is what 'normal'

feels like, I think to myself, amazed at what I have achieved.

All my life, I had struggled with a vague sense that something was different about me. I felt inferior, inadequate, undisciplined, and hopelessly disorganized —feelings that have, at one time or another, been reinforced by others in my life.

"Donna, can't you ever be on time?"

"I couldn't live in this clutter."

"How can you not know where your daughters' birth certificates are?"

"Maybe you're just one of those people who can't stay organised."

I had gotten used to feeling tired before I even got out of bed, dreading every new day and its various obligations. I was exhausted, struggling at work and home with my kids. It took every ounce of physical, mental, emotional, and spiritual strength to live my life — until I finally met someone who listened to my story and gave me a chance to do something about it.

He didn't hand me a planner or a book on organisation. He didn't lecture me on slothfulness or give me parenting advice. He handed me a prescription.

"Take this and see what happens," he said. "I think you have adult ADD." He was the first person ever to believe me when I said that there was something wrong beyond depression or a fundamentally disorganised personality. I had always sensed that there was a part of me that could be structured, that could be organised, that could function with ease. I just didn't know where it was or how to access it.

A new mom…

As we pulled into a gas station one day, another car pulled in front of us. The driver was shouting and cursing. At the station, I walked over to her. "Hey, I'm sorry if I irritated you," I said. "I'm taking my kids to school, we were talking, and maybe I didn't give you enough space."

The woman calmed down noticeably and shook her head. "No, it's my fault," she said. "I'm tired this morning and I got mad. Don't worry about it." As I got back in our car, my oldest daughter, Zoë, stared at me, eyes wide open.

"Mama," she said eagerly, "I can't believe how nice you were!" How embarrassing it was to realise what a jerk your kids thought you were, in the throes of daily ADD-related irritability. I grinned. "You've got a new mama, girls!" I said as we continued on our way.

In the past, a situation like that would have caused me to erupt. I'd fuss and fume and blare my horn. I used to think I had a problem with anger. Now I know that my nerves were just stretched to their limits, and things that rolled off other peoples' backs were intolerable to me.

Our life has slowed down at home. We eat in more often, and my girls enjoy my cooking. I'm not trying to do 15 other things while making dinner anymore, so I don't end up burning it. I've also come up with my own system to organise my cabinets — and it works!

Because I now understand that I have a disorder that requires me to do things a little differently, I do them without feeling that I'm stupid or lazy. What I've discovered about myself is just the opposite: I can be highly organised and disciplined if I let myself be. My medicine has calmed something down inside of me, allowed me to take a deep breath and live at a slower pace.

Don't give up on being able to live a normal life because there is hope.

References

1. ADHD Awareness Month (2023). 7 Facts You Need to Know About ADHD. Retrieved Nov 14, 2023, from https://www.adhdawarenessmonth.org/7-facts-about-adhd/

2. ADHD Institute (2023). Burden of ADHD, Epidemiology. Retrieved November 14, 2023, from https://adhd-institute.com/burden-of-adhd

3. American Psychiatric Association. Diagnostic and Statistical Manual of Mental Disorders, Fifth Edition. 2013.topics

4. Centers for Disease Control and Prevention (May 2016). Attention-Deficit/Hyperactivity Disorder (ADHD). Retrieved June 16, 2016, from http://www.cdc.gov/ncbddd/adhd/data.html

5. HealthLine (March 2019). ADHD By The Numbers: Facts, Statistics and You. Retrieved November 14, 2023, from https://www.healthline.com/health/adhd/facts-statistics-infographic

6. National Institute of Mental Health (2023). Attention Deficit Hyperactivity Disorder. Retrieved November 14,

2023, from
https://www.nimh.nih.gov/health/topics/attention-deficit-hyperactivity-disorder-adhd

7. Psychiatry Advisor (March 2015). Estimates of ADHD Prevalence Worldwide Differ Significantly. Retrieved June 15, 2016, from
https://www.psychiatryadvisor.com/home/topics/adhd/estimates-of-adhd-prevalence-worldwide-differ-significantly/

www.ingramcontent.com/pod-product-compliance
Lightning Source LLC
Chambersburg PA
CBHW080427030426
42335CB00020B/2624